Meditation for Beginners, Without the Woo-Woo

A Practical Guide for the Everyday Person

Clive Smit

ISBN: 978-0-473-33823-7

Cover Design: Clive Smit
Interior Design: Clive Smit
Book Cover Photograph: Steve Johnson on Flickr Creative Commons

Contact the author at futurepastpodcast@gmail.com

DEDICATION

To my angel, with your encouragement I have had the courage to walk on water.

To my children, Ethan, Laykin, Mila & Kingston, you keep me young and fill me with inspiration every day.

BONUS CONTENT:

If you'd like to receive a guided audio meditation for free then simply go to http://futurepastpodcast.com/get-your-free-meditation-bonus/

PLEASE REVIEW THE BOOK ON AMAZON

It would be greatly appreciated if you could place an honest review for this book on Amazon. Your review helps others to know if this book is right for them.

CONTENTS

	DEFINITIONS	i
1	INTRODUCTION	1
2	SEVEN BENEFITS OF MEDITATION	5
3	MIND-SET	10
4	BREATH	13
5	YOUR FIRST MEDITATION, STEP BY STEP	16
6	SEVEN MEDITATION TECHNIQUES	21
7	DEEP BREATHING	26
8	FIVE COMMON OBSTACLES	30
9	TYPES OF MEDITATION	33
10	FAQ'S	36
11	FURTHER RESOURCES	40
12	IN CLOSING	43
	ABOUT THE AUTHOR	**45**

DEFINITIONS

Meditation:

The mastering of one's mind through the practice of being present.

Woo-woo:

An unfounded or ludicrous belief. Any belief that is not founded on evidence.

(From the Urban Dictionary)

Return to Breath:

To return your focus to your breath by paying attention to your incoming and outgoing breath on the rim of your nose..

ONE

INTRODUCTION

"The real Meditation practice is how we live our lives from moment to moment to moment."

- *Jon Kabat-Zinn*

Although meditation is becoming increasingly popular I can remember growing up and thinking it was just an Eastern woo-woo practice. Whenever movies showed people who meditated they were eccentric people whose homes were filled with incense and who wore hippy clothing. That definitely was not who I wanted to be and because of this I ignored this extremely valuable practice that has been around for millennia.

To be honest the only reason that I gave meditation a go is because of the value that Tim Ferriss (of the 4-Hour Work Week fame) placed on the practice. This made me curious and then I discovered that there was an impressive amount of uber successful people that not only practiced meditation but also noted it as one of the most important practices that contributes to their success in life. Below is what a few of these people had to say:

Ray Dalio, Billionare**,** CEO and founder of Bridgewater Associates "Meditation, more than any other factors have been the secrets to whatever success I've had"

"Meditation lead to openness, to freedom, where a kind of intuition just comes through. You could step back and put things in perspective. It doesn't lessen your emotions. The emotions are the same, but you can step back and say, "I'm not going to be controlled by that emotion," and I think it then helps to see things at a higher level,"

Ramani Ayer, former CEO of The Hartford – an insurance company that rose to the Fortune 100 under his leadership. He is presently on the board of directors for the XL Group.

Meditation has helped me to consistently raise my performance levels."

"In terms of my professional life, meditation has helped me to consistently raise my performance levels. It has helped me cope with the stresses and strains of life. And I believe very strongly that the practice of meditation has helped me to maintain a steady state of mind — it has given me equanimity no matter what happens."

Dr. Oz, cardiothoracic surgeon, author and television personality

"It's like, imagine the ripples on top of an ocean. And I'm in a rowboat, reactively dealing with the waves and water coming into my boat. What I need to do is dive into the deeper solace, the calmness beneath the surface."

Dr. Fred Travis, leading Neuroscientist and author

"What I think meditation is doing is erasing that line between challenge and stress. You can take on increasingly more and more challenge without it becoming stressful. I think some of that is because you never have the perception that it's too much; you never have the perception that this experience is going to overtake you."

Ellen DeGeneres, comedian, television host, actress, writer, and producer.

"It feels good. Kinda like when you have to shut your computer down, just sometimes when it goes crazy, you just shut it down and when you turn it on, it's okay again. That's what meditation is to me."

Jerry Seinfeld, stand up comedian and actor

"With Seinfeld, I was doing a TV series in which I was the star of the show, the executive producer of the show, the head writer, in charge of casting and editing, for 24 episodes on network television, not cable – for nine years! And I'm just a normal guy. And that was not a normal situation to be in… So I meditated every day. And that's how I survived the nine years."

Clint Eastwood, film director, actor & producer

"I've been using it for almost 40 years now – and I think it's a great tool for anyone to have, to be able to utilize as a tool for stress. Stress, of course, comes with almost every business."

Martin Scorsese, director, screenwriter and producer

"It's difficult to describe the effect it has had on my life. I can only mention may-be a few words: calm, clarity, a balance, and at times — a recognition.
For me, meditation has made a difference."

Sheryl Crow, singer & songwriter

"One of the things – and this comes from someone who was highly self-critical and a type-A personality – that has changed my life is meditating."

Sir Paul McCartney, singer-songwriter, multi-instrumentalist, and composer.

"Meditation is a lifelong gift. It's something you can call on at any time. I think it's a great thing."

When I saw that this wide range of successful people from multiple fields experienced benefits from meditation, I decided to dip my toe into the waters of meditation. It's amazing the prejudice that you can have when you haven't experienced something for yourself. Now, are there some meditation practices that aren't for me? There sure are. But I found out first hand that meditation doesn't have to have any woo-woo. In fact, the science behind meditation is really solid.

Meditation isn't a silver bullet to fix everything in your life. It is a really brilliant tool to master your mind and to learn how to be present in the moment that you're in. Along with the 10 successful people above, I too highly recommend the practice of meditation because of the benefits that I have personally experienced. As we get into the book I'll share these benefits with you.

What You'll Get From This Book

I am someone who doesn't want to spend hours on end learning about a subject before I get stuck in doing. In fact, I believe that we should generally set a limit of 30 minutes of learning before getting stuck in and trying something out (we've all met people who have spent tens if not hundreds of hours learning and have never taken any action!)
So I give you a no fluff guarantee. I know that you're a busy and productive person who just needs to get on with it, so I promise to remove the fluff and just get to the point.

In this book you'll discover the seven personal benefits of practicing meditation and I'll equip with you with the mind-set and practical steps to get meditating today. Also included will be some common obstacles that people encounter, FAQ's and further resources that I believe will be beneficial for you on your meditative journey.

TWO

SEVEN BENEFITS OF MEDITATION

"Take care of your body. It's the only place you have to live."
- Jim Rohn

So just before we get into the nitty-gritty of how to meditate without the woo-woo, I wanted to share seven benefits of meditating regularly.

Benefit 1: A Sharpened Focus

Focus is the key to success in life. The difference between the ultra productive and the average person comes down to this one principal: Focus!

Studies have shown that what separates the top 3%, 20% and the rest of the CEO's is the number of priorities that they focus on.

The top 3% have only 1-2 priorities, while the top 20% have 3-5 priorities and the rest have 5-15 priorities.

We have all experienced the debilitating feeling of being pulled in all directions. It weakens our focus and when we get to the end of the day we realize that we haven't accomplished anything significant.

We all know what it is like to be hit on every side by demands for our attention: Our spouse wants attention, our children want attention, our boss and managers want attention. Our email screams out. Our Facebook, Pinterest and Twitter accounts call to us. Advertisers want our attention and bombard us with 16 000 messages a day. And on top of the outward requests and calls for our attention we are also inundated with our own thoughts.

Each 24 hour day we have 70 000 thoughts (we are thinking even while sleeping). Now that is a lot of thoughts! A 24 hour day is made up of 86 400 seconds. So that equates to 1 thought every 1.2 seconds!

This is where meditation is a great tool to teach us focus. Study after study has shown that meditation helps people to focus their attention and sustain it, even during the most boring of tasks. Meditation is a workout for your mind. And that focus can bring massive results to your productivity!

Benefit 2: Boosting Your Creativity

Creativity is also essential for success. The problem is that most people don't give their minds the space it needs to be creative.

Creativity helps you to problem solve and turn obstacles into opportunity.

Albert Einstein practiced what is called 'hard thinking' and 'soft thinking'. He would pour over his calculations, engage in deep conversations and do 'hard thinking' work. Then he would switch to doing an activity such as playing the violin or sailing where he could get lost in his pleasurable pursuit.

Einstein realized that while enjoying himself in these pursuits that his mind was subconsciously working on the problems and he would receive insights at unexpected times. This was the result of his 'soft thinking'.

Thomas Edison had a similar practice where he would take strolls between laboratories to 'soft think'. I am sure that you have personally experienced insights coming to you while you're in the shower, or driving, etc.

Meditation allows our minds the space to move into soft thinking that can bring much needed insight into your day. I would regularly take a lunch break to meditate and was always pleased I took the time out. I came back into the second half of the day fresh, creative and productive.

Benefit 3: Overcome Stress

If there is one common experience that people have today it is stress. And while there is eustress (a good stress) that helps us to be productive, most of us are dealing with negative stress. When we are stressed out our immune system is weakened, our body's cells are tired, we experience negative thoughts, we demand more from ourselves, we lack concentration and we make more mistakes.

A large factor of the stress that we face is the desire to get things done combined with our fear that we won't get those things done. As well as meditation here are some things you can do to alleviate your stress:

- Create Margin (don't fill up every single second of your day.)
- Write down a to-do list (itemize the tasks that you absolutely have to get done for that day only) and STOP once you've completed the list.
- Use Parkinson's Law (which states that – psychologically – work will expand to fill the time allotted to it.) Shorten the time you allot for completing tasks, stop procrastinating and just get it done.
- Practice the 80/20 Rule (80% of our productivity comes from 20% of our work – so focus on doing that 20%!)

Practicing meditation with the above will see your stress levels come into the healthy zone that makes you more productive.

Meditation has been shown to reduce both the physical and emotional response to stress. Studies have shown that after eight weeks of meditation practice there is more electrical activity in the left frontal lobe region of the brain – which is an area of the brain that tends to be more active in optimistic people.

Meditation allows you to focus your attention and eliminate the stream of thoughts that crowd your mind causing you stress. It also deeply relaxes your body. It is this double whammy that makes meditation such an effective practice for reducing your stress levels.

Benefit 4: A Healthier body

Some of the benefits to your body are:

- Lowers your blood pressure (In one study 2/3rds of high blood pressure patients who started meditating could stop taking their blood pressure medication!)
- Improves your blood circulation
- Lowers your heart rate
- Perspire less
- Gives you a lower respiratory rate
- Lowers your blood cortisol levels
- Increases your energy levels
- Lowers the level of your blood lactate, which reduces anxiety attacks
- Reduces tension related pain
- Increases your serotonin which improves your mood
- Improves your immune system

Benefit 5: Energizes Your Mind

Regular meditation leads to:

- Neuroplasticity (The brains ability to reorganize itself by forming new neural connections. This helps the brain respond to new situations or to changes in one's environment.)
- Develop thicker cortical walls (Which means your brain ages slower. Your cortical thickness is also associated with decision-making, attention and memory.)
- Reduces symptoms of depression as effectively as antidepressants.

Benefit 6: We Learn to Live in the Present

Another wonderful benefit of meditation is learning presence. It is common now that much of our time is spent on devises. Even when we are home we can find ourselves 'at the office' and when we're at the office social media and everyone else's agendas are interrupting us. When we're talking to people we're checking our watch and looking over people's shoulders thinking of all the other things that we need to get done. We totally miss out on the moment and all the opportunities it wants to present us.

Meditation teaches one how to be present in the moment and that benefit is priceless.

Benefit 7: Opens Your Heart

Often we spend so much time running on the treadmill of life that we don't stop to address what is going on emotionally. And emotions are like a cork, you can push them down, but eventually they'll popup and usually they'll come up with force!

We tend to believe that we can simply hide our emotions and that they won't have an impact on our day-to-day interactions. The truth is that people can sense what we are feeling. And on top of that, we react differently in the same circumstances depending on our emotional state.

Unresolved emotions such as: anger, disappointment, loneliness, emptiness, anxiety, etc will affect those around us and ourselves. Meditation helps you to quite down enough to acknowledge those emotions. And awareness is the first step to dealing with any issue.

You also gain a much clearer understanding of your own thought processes, which means you can then have more control over what you think.

THREE

MIND-SET

"My greatest challenge has been to change the mindset of people. Mindsets play strange tricks on us. We see things the way our minds have instructed our eyes to see."

- *Muhammad Yunus*

As we begin the journey to discovering meditation there are three important mind-sets that we must carry. If you have these mind-sets then you'll find meditation to be an enjoyable practice. Let's look at each of these mind-sets.

Mind-set 1: Everything is an Experiment

A lot of people in the world today do not want to try anything new for fear of failure. They'd rather not try anything than fail. A much better mind-set is to see everything as an experiment. You can't fail by trying something. Experiments are all about giving things a go and finding out what works by trial and error. It's having the same attitude as Thomas Edison when he famously said, *"I have not failed. I've just found 10 000 ways that won't work."*

This is the mind-set that all children carry as they experiment with the world around them. This mind-set sets you free to enjoy the world around you as you continually experiment.

Let's be honest. Just about everyone has heard that meditation is beneficial. But most people have never experimented with it. You are taking action and that's what separates you from everyone else. So give yourself a pat on the back!

Experimenting also allows you to find what works for you. We are all different and we certainly were not made with the same cookie cutter. What might work for one person will not necessarily be a good fit for you. When you are discovering meditation you have to find your own path and realize that there is no right or wrong way to do it, just your way. And the only way to discover it is to experiment with different techniques.

Mind-set 2: Meditation is Active

Many people believe that meditation is a passive practice where you sit in a state of thoughtless peacefulness. The practice of meditation is a very active process. It's a workout for your mind! In meditation you are training your mind in the art of focus.

Mind-set 3: Meditation is About Returning Your Focus

Typically in the beginning, especially the more driven you are, you will find yourself frustrated when meditating. This is because almost instantaneously after sitting down to meditate your mind will sprint off in all directions. And if you hold the mind-set that meditation is about perfection, then you will become angry and frustrated.

Instead we need to approach meditation with the mindset that it is all about returning to your focus. (Often the object of focus is your breath. To return to your breath you simply bring your focus back to your breathing, noting the incoming and outgoing breath on the rim of your nose.) So when the thoughts come, there is no need to get frustrated. Just realize that our minds are like a wild stallion that you are seeking to tame over time. It's bucking, it's pulling against any kind of line you put on it, but ultimately the circles get smaller and smaller. Your return to your focus gets easier and easier. As long as you are returning to your focus you're doing just fine.

With the right mind-sets under your belt you will be able to experience the pleasure of meditation. Now you'll be in the position to discover just why this practice has been around for millennia.

FOUR

BREATH

"For breath is life, and if you breathe well you will live long on earth."

- *Sanskrit Proverb*

The very centerpiece of meditation is your breath. Breath is essential to life. It is the first thing we do when we are born and it is the last thing we do before we leave this earth. In between that time we take about half a billion breathes.

We may not realize this but the mind, body and breath are interconnected. Our breathing is influenced by our thoughts. Likewise our thoughts and physiology can be influenced by our breathing. For instance, have you noticed that when you are raging mad that your breath is quick, short, sharp and forceful?

And have you ever seen someone who is having an asthma attack? They panic and their breathing becomes quicker and shallower which worsens the situation. A parent, family member or friend can remedy this when they come alongside and get the person to focus on just taking deep and long breathes. And in no time they come right as rain.

Now, while you may not be asthmatic, the fact is that most of us breathe very shallow due to the massive amounts of stress that we carry.

Learning to breathe properly brings tremendous benefits such as:

- Releasing up to 70% of the bodies toxins
- Muscle relaxation
- Increased energy levels
- Lower blood pressure
- Elevating mood and reducing feelings of stress, anxiety and depression

The second key benefit of breathing in meditation is that it helps us focus our attention. Jon Kabat-Zinn, author of 'Wherever You Go, There You Are', says the following about breathing, *"It helps to have a focus for your attention, an anchor line to tether you to the present moment and to guide you back when the mind wanders. The breath serves this purpose… Bringing awareness to our breathing we remind ourselves that we are here now."*

Meditative breathing teaches the mind and body to let go; like the breath, troubling thoughts and feelings come and go, they come and they go. As you learn to quiet the mind by paying attention to your breathing, distractions lose their power to disrupt your focus and disturb your mind.

Think of your nose as a lighthouse. If you get lost in a sea of thought… simply come back to your breathing. Always back to breathing. In and out; nice and slow and steady.

Two Types of Breathing

The first type of breathing is the standard for meditative practice. It is simply a focus on your breath without any attempt to alter or control it. If your breathing is out of sync it will eventually come back to where it should be.

The second type is a deep breathing. Here the focus is not only on the breath but also on breathing the 'right' way. Most people breathe from the top half of their lungs. Deep breathing teaches you to fill your lungs entirely. You should feel the air filling your chest and abdomen.

The added benefits of deep breathing meditation are:

- It strengthens the lungs
- It massages your organs
- It improves your nervous system
- It increases your digestion of food
- It strengthens the immune system
- And it helps release muscle tension

Now that you know the benefits of meditation, of having the right mind-set and the importance of your breath, you are now ready to get your nose out of the book and try out your first meditation.

FIVE

YOUR FIRST MEDITATION, STEP BY STEP

"Meditation is a lifelong process. Give it a try. As you get deeper and more disciplined into the process, you'll get deeper and more disciplined in your mind and life."

- *Brendon Burchard*

Congratulations on making it this far! I am sure that you are looking forward to trying meditation out for yourself. In this chapter I'll walk you through your first meditation step by step.

Preparing the space

There are two types of space that you must prepare. The first is the space in your calendar. When are you going to be meditating? This is an important space to create as habits are formed most easily when there is a consistent time and physical space.

Some people meditate twice a day. Some once. Others meditate at multiple times throughout the day. The important thing for now is that you simply make the 'time' space for meditating.

Many people choose the beginning of the day and or the end of the day. Just find a time that works for you, provides you with the quiet and privacy that you'll need so that you aren't constantly interrupted.

The second space that you'll need to create is the physical one. Make sure that interruptions are prevented. You may need to tell others in your household that this is your time and not to interrupt you. Put your phone away (unless you're using a meditation app) and on silent. Make sure you have chosen a quiet part of the house. Some people like to have music in the background. Just do what works for you.

Posture

Choose a comfortable and upright chair and use a cushion in the small of your back. Sit in a dignified manner, with your back upright (alert but relaxed) and imagine a string pulling up your head. Take a second to tune in to your posture and ask if you are tenser than you need to be. Sit straighter, loosen your shoulders, arms and stomach. Give a sigh and release that tension.

Have your feet flat on the floor with your hands on your thighs. You can also place one hand inside the other in a ball. Whatever is comfortable, do that.

Now have a gentle smile. You'll be amazed what a difference a smile and sitting dignified makes. Your body is sending cues to your mind and vice versa.

Your posture is important as it creates a body attitude, effects your mood, hormone levels and energy.

Have you ever seen a depressed person with their head held up high? Have you ever seen a person who lacks confidence standing tall? Perhaps there is more to the old cliché than we realize that says 'keep your chin up'.

When you have good posture there is an increase in your testosterone levels (associated with self confidence) and a decrease in cortisol levels (the stress hormone).

Good posture also affects your energy levels as your muscles are being used more efficiently to keep you erect. When muscles are overworked due to poor posture your muscles will spasm, draining your vitality.

Roger Sperns, PhD, who is a Nobel Prize winner for his research on the brain says, *"The more mechanically distorted a person is, the less energy is available for thinking, metabolism and healing."*

The PMR Meditation

The body scan is a very common meditation technique. There are many versions of it, but the one I will get you to start with is called Progressive Muscle Relaxation. It is one of the oldest Western meditation exercises dating back to the 1930's. In this meditation you scan through the body, making it tense for a moment and then relax. This meditation is a great starting point as it teaches you how your muscles feel when they are tensed and how they feel when they are relaxed. Ultimately, this awareness is all you will need in your meditative journey. Once you have trained yourself as to how your body feels when it is relaxed then your body will gravitate to that state of being whenever you give it a chance.

Step 1:

Get comfortable in your chair. Take a few deep breaths.

Step 2:

Close your eyes and take a few more deep breaths.

Step 3:

In this step you will scan your feet, legs and hips, taking note of how they feel.

With each breath tense an area, breathing in and out, and then release, breathing in and out.

Then move on to the next area. First your feet, then your calves, legs and hips.

Step 4:

Scan your belly and lower back. Tensing and releasing.

Tense - breathe in and out.

Release - breathe in and out.

Notice the feelings and sensations.

Step 5:

Scan your diaphragm (at the bottom of your rib cage) and solar plexus (just below your sternum). Feel the movement of the lower ribs.

Tense - breathe in and out.
Release - breathe in and out.

Step 6:

Now scan your chest and upper back.

Tense - breathe in and out.
Release - breathe in and out.

Step 7:

Then scan your neck, shoulders, arms and hands.

Tense - breathe in and out.
Release - breathe in and out.

Step 8:

Now for your scalp and forehead.

Tense (frown) - breathe in and out.
Release -breathe in and out.

Step 9:

Now tense your whole body -breathe in and out.

Release - breathe in and out.
Now sit for a few moments breathing in and out.

Step 10:

Finely, take a few deep breaths and open your eyes.

Take a last few deep breaths and just take it all in for a minute.

After Your Meditations

I have found that straight after your time of meditation is a great time to practice Gratitude Journaling and a review of your day's to-do list and priorities. This is not a common meditation teaching, but I have just found it to be a helpful add-on to my meditations.

To-Do List

To-Do lists have been around for a long time. It amazes me how many people don't have a to-do list. When we leave everything in our head this uses up a lot of mental energy. Not to mention it means that you end up forgetting things.

Take some time to brainstorm all that must be accomplished. Write down absolutely everything that you can think of. Make sure to include your business and personal items in here. This is your master list.

Then at the beginning of the week, you can draw from the list everything that must be accomplished for this week. You can also add any items to your weekly to-do list that weren't on your master list.Now each day you must write a fresh list (using your weekly list). These are the items that you MUST accomplish for that day. And remember, once you have ticked everything off on your list... you can STOP! This practice helps to create the needed margin in your life.

If you want to take your personal productivity to the next level then I would highly recommend David Allan's book Getting Things Done. I can also recommend Rory Vaden's new book called Procrastinate on Purpose. You can find both those books at http://futurepastpodcast.com/meditation-resources/

Your Gratitude Journal

You can use a scrapbook and write down:

- 3 things that you are grateful for in your personal life
- 3 Things that you are grateful for in your value exchange (work) life
- 3 Things that you are grateful for about yourself

Or you can purchase the Five Minute Journal at http://futurepastpodcast.com/meditation-resources/

Let me reiterate, gratitude journaling isn't a woo-woo practice. Like meditation it teaches you to focus. And this focus will elevate your thinking and actions and it will definitely help you to add value in other people's lives.

SIX

SEVEN MEDITATION TECHNIQUES

"Life wants you to touch, taste and see the grandeur of the world's unfathomable variety."

Bryant McGill

There are many types of meditation. So which one is right for you? You'll have to experiment to find that out. And there is nothing better than doing something new. Variety is certainly the spice of life! Here are a few techniques for you to give a whirl:

The Breathing Technique

In this meditation practice you simply focus on your breath. You are not trying to direct it. It is simply your focal point.

If your mind starts to wonder, simply return to your breath.

Some people like to count while they breathe. Count one and breathe in. Count two and breathe out. Continue this until you reach ten and start again at one.

When your mind wanders, simply return to the count of one. Eventually you'll be able to follow your breathing without counting.

Some people like to use this technique as it connects the mind to your breath.

The Body Scan

This is a very popular meditation technique that can promote body awareness, stress awareness and relaxation.

As we take a 'tour' of your body by scanning each part, try and bring an attitude of curiosity, as if you are investigating your body for the first time. Become aware of any and all sensations that are present, such as heat, cold, pressure, tightness, tingling, etc. If you do come across an area that is tense, see if you can relax it and allow it to soften. If it doesn't, just simply notice how it feels and move on. You may also become aware of thoughts or emotions as you scan through various areas. Simply note these and return to the scan. If you do not feel any sensations, thoughts or emotions, that's fine, just move along to the next part of the scan.

Begin by bringing attention to your breathing.

Start the scan with your head, neck and then shoulders. Then move on to your arms and hands. Then your upper and lower back, chest, stomach and buttocks. And then your hips, legs and feet.

Finally, take note of your body as a whole. Take a minute to just sit and feel this expansive awareness.

The Walk By Technique

This is a very simple meditation technique used to improve mood and concentration.

Sit on a park bench or in any public place and direct your eyes forward as strangers walk by.

The idea is to avoid looking at the passers-by even if they look interesting. You just let them walk by. You notice them, but you keep your mind focused on not watching them, not following them.

And as always, practice your breathing.

Movement Meditation

Movement meditation mixes movement with meditation. This can be done while walking, doing Tai Chi, washing the dishes, etc.

Paying attention to your body while you are moving will help you to simply enjoy being alive.

Here is an example using walking meditation:

Before starting the walk, spend a few moments becoming aware of your body. Become aware of all the subtle movements involved in keeping your body balanced. Take some deep breaths.

As you begin walking start at a relaxed but normal pace. Pay attention to the sensations in your body as you walk. It is natural to find your attention being drawn towards the sights as you walk but simply bring your attention back to what is going on internally.

The idea is to have your attention on the physical experience of walking.

Notice in detail how your body feels as you walk. Notice the feelings in your feet, calves, knees, and thighs, the swinging of your arms, your back, shoulders and neck (you may even want to exaggerate a few of the movements so that you can get a feel of what is going on in that area.)

When you come to the end of the walk spend a few minutes just standing. Notice what it is like to no longer be in motion. Take note again of the complex balancing act that keeps you standing. Take a last few deep breaths.

Visualization

Visualization is a powerful tool that expands your creativity.

Celebrities like Jim Carey, Barbra Streisand, Jack Canfield (Chicken Soup for the Soul), Arnold Schwarzenegger, professional athletes and many others are known to practice visual meditation.

Visualization can be used to create calming or peaceful images that set up a great space from which to meditate from. Visualization can also be used to envision success or for keeping calm under pressure filled environments.

To begin, focus your mind by paying attention to your breath.

After a few minutes generate your image. The more detailed you make it the better. Make the picture as sensual as possible, taking note of sights, sounds, smells, touch and taste. Also take note of how you feel in that space.

The more often you visualize, the easier it will be to return to that space.

Nature Meditation

Being out in nature is a great way to meditate. You can either meditate with your eyes closed or open.

Begin with placing your attention on your breathing.

Once you feel focused, you can then expand your awareness to your environment. Take in all that the environment has to offer. Feel the temperature of the air on your skin, the feeling of the breeze and the sun. Notice the sounds around you. Listen to the symphony of nature.

If your mind wanders, just bring it back to the experience of nature.

As you meditate, you can see where your attention is naturally drawn, or you can purposefully scan for different experiences. You can also focus in on a single experience and notice it in greater detail. Don't analyze or label it, just notice it.

You can also tune in to the feelings that being in nature bring.

My favorite is to sit under the stars and just take the vastness of it all in.

Mindfulness Meditation

Mindfulness meditation encourages one to observe wandering thoughts as they drift through your consciousness. You are not getting involved with the thoughts or judging them, you are simply aware of them. You aren't engaging the thoughts but rather you are keeping them at an arms length.

In this meditation practice you develop an awareness of how your thoughts and feelings tend to move in particular patterns.

This practice is great for teaching you to relate differently to your distractions and increase your ability to concentrate and focus.

It can be useful to begin this meditation with a body scan.

Once you have completed this, while keeping some attention on your breath and the environment, you can take note of your individual thoughts and the themes of thoughts that come to mind. Note how this changes depending on your energy levels and moods.

It is not uncommon to have a barrage of thoughts. That's ok. Just note the thoughts in a non-judgmental way by saying to yourself, "Thoughts." (Think of it like a weather report, 'Thinking has just occurred in this vicinity.')

Once you have noted the thoughts just let them drift on.

If at any point you get lost in the thoughts, simply return your focus to your anchor - your breath. No need to judge or get upset.

Once you've noted the general state of your thoughts you can then gently change the state of your consciousness by introducing compassion when feeling depressed, goodwill when feeling angry and appreciation when feeling dissatisfied.

I have introduced you to seven meditation techniques. There are of course many more but these seven are a great place to start. You will find that you connect with some of the techniques much more naturally. Use these more natural techniques as your core meditation practices. However, it is always good to mix things up every now and again and practice a totally different technique as this broadens your meditative experience.

SEVEN

DEEP BREATHING

"If you want to conquer the anxiety of life, live in the moment, live in the breath."

Amit Ray

While meditating, the general idea is not to overly control your breathing. Deep breathing is a great practice to have alongside or integrated into your meditative practice. It can be practiced before or with your meditation, or even on its own at various times throughout the day as needed.

When you are experiencing stress, your nervous system triggers the body's ancient fight-or-flight response, giving you a burst of energy to respond to the perceived danger. Your breathing becomes shallow and rapid. This can make you feel lightheaded, which is a common symptom when you feel anxious or frustrated.

At the same time your body releases adrenaline, which increases your blood pressure and pulse rate.

With deep breathing you can reverse these symptoms instantly and create a sense of calm in your body and mind.

Deep breathing has been found to be helpful in treating depression, anxiety, post-traumatic stress disorder, chronic destructive pulmonary disease and asthma.

4 Deep Breathing Exercises

A regular daily practice of deep breathing is one of the best tools for improving your health and wellbeing. Performing one of these deep breathing techniques twice daily for only three to five minutes can produce extraordinary long-term benefits. You can also use them any time that you are feeling stressed or notice that your breathing has become constricted. By training your body with a regular practice of deep breathing, you will begin to breathe more effectively even without concentrating on it.

Complete Belly Breath

For a general practice of deep breathing you can place one hand on your belly, relaxing your abdominal muscles. Slowly inhale through the nose, bringing the air to the bottom of your lungs. Once your collarbones have risen and you can no longer take in any more air (you should have felt your abdomen rise) then pause for a moment before gently exhaling. At the end, contract your abdominal muscles slightly to push residual air out of the bottom of your lungs.

Repeat this for three to five minutes.

Alternate Nostril Breathing

This is a great practice for when you are feeling nervous or ungrounded. This exercise will immediately help you to feel calmer.

Hold your right thumb over your right nostril and inhale deeply through your left nostril.

At the peak of your inhalation, close off your left nostril with your index finger, lift your right thumb, and then exhale smoothly through your right nostril.

After a full exhalation, inhale through the right nostril, closing it off with your right thumb at the peak of your inhalation, lift your index finger and exhale smoothly through your left nostril.

Continue with this practice for three to five minutes alternating your breath through each nostril. Your breathing should be effortless, with your mind gently observing the inflow and outflow of breath.

Ocean's Breath

This is a great practice for when you feel angry, irritated or frustrated. This will immediately settle and soothe your mind.

Take an inhalation that is slightly deeper than normal. With your mouth closed, exhale through your nose while constricting your throat muscles. If you are doing this correctly, you should sound like waves on the ocean.

Another way to get the hang of this practice is to try exhaling the sound 'haaaaaaah' with your with your mouth open. Now make a similar sound with your mouth closed, feeling the outflow of air through your nasal passages.

Once you have mastered this on the outflow, use the same method for the inflow breath, gently constricting your throat as you inhale.

Energizing Breath

This is a great practice for when you are feeling blue or sluggish. This practice will give you an immediate surge of energy and invigorate your mind.

Note: do not practice this if you are pregnant or have uncontrolled hypertension, epilepsy/seizures, panic disorder, hernia, gastric ulcer, glaucoma, or vertigo. Use caution if you have an underlying lung disease.

Begin by relaxing your shoulders and take a few deep, full breaths from your abdomen.

Now start exhaling forcefully through your nose, followed by forceful deep inhalations at the rate of one second per cycle.

Your breathing is entirely from your diaphragm, keeping your head, neck, shoulders and chest relatively still while your belly moves in and out.

Start by doing a round of ten breaths, then breathe naturally and notice the sensations in your body.

After fifteen to thirty seconds begin the next round with twenty breaths.

Finally after pausing for another thirty seconds, complete a third round of thirty breaths.

Beginners are advised to take a break between rounds. Stay tuned to your body during the process. If you are feeling lightheaded or uncomfortable, then stop for a few moments before resuming in a less intense manner.

EIGHT

FIVE COMMON OBSTACLES

"Success is to be measured not so much by the position that one has reached in life as by the obstacles which he has overcome."

Booker T Washington

Now that you have experienced a taste of meditation for yourself, you may be wandering why more people are not practicing meditation. Well, as with anything worthwhile, it's not easy going all the time. There are many obstacles that must be overcome. We'll look at five of the most common obstacles that the majority of people face at one time or another.

Obstacle 1: I Don't Have the Time

This is possibly the most common obstacle that challenges those who would try to make meditation a habitual practice. This obstacle is connected to the plague of busyness that has gripped our world today.

However, being the effective and productive person that you are, you know the power of prioritizing the things that are most important.

I love the quote from Jim Rohn that says, *"We must all suffer from one of two pains: the pain of discipline or the pain of regret. The difference is discipline weighs ounces while regret weighs tons."*

We can either be disciplined about prioritizing the most important things into our day or we'll end up doing everything except for the important things.

Another reason we don't prioritize is that we feel guilty about investing time in the most important of activities, as these are the activities that don't cry out for our attention. What we need to do is give ourselves the emotional permission to do what matters most. Rory Vaden's book Procrastinate on Purpose is an excellent resource for learning to give yourself the needed emotional permission to focus on what is most important. You can find Rory's book at http://futurepastpodcast.com/meditation-resources/

Obstacle 2: I Can't Stop Thinking

This is another very common obstacle for those who meditate, and it's not just an obstacle for beginners. The good news is that it does get easier with time.

Many people approach meditating with an idealism that says it will be perfect. But this is the wrong mind-set altogether. Remember, meditation is simply a return to your object of focus. When you realize that you have been distracted, just bring your attention back.

The trouble that most beginners get into is that they make a big deal about the intruding thoughts. They start to focus on it more and more, feeding it and causing it to take up more of your attention. So just don't feed it. Simply acknowledge that it is there and carry on.

Some people simply name the distraction. This moves it off centre stage and as you return focus to your breath the thought is then able to move on. Just like a cloud that covers the sun. It may block your focus for a moment but just relax and let it move on.

Obstacle 3: I'm Restless

Just the thought of sitting still for active people and natural go getters can be disconcerting! But with practice this will be come normal for you. Like a car that shifts into neutral it can take a little while for the engine to return to idle.

Your self-talk is important. It can either lead you to get frustrated with yourself and the process or it can encourage you to be patient with yourself and the process.

Obstacle 4: I'm Nodding Off

Nodding off can happen especially if you are getting up early to meditate or if you are doing it before going to bed.

If you're waking up early I would recommend that you don't meditate until 10-15 minutes after getting out of bed. Have a shower or stretch. Splash your face with water. Don't drink coffee yet but you can have a cup of water (hot or cold) with half of a fresh lemon's juice squeezed into it (trust me, it's just as good as a cup of coffee!) This will have you in the alert zone that you will need to be in to meditate.

If you are doing it before bed I'd suggest not meditating in your bed… unless you want to fall asleep.

Obstacle 5: Feelings of Discomfort

Because most people are walking around under constant stress (and even experience tightened muscles and grinding of ones teeth in their sleep), when our bodies do finally get the chance to relax we can sometimes experience some discomfort. This is because when we are tense we produce adrenalin and endorphins – natural opiates – that tend to numb our body. As you relax you begin to feel the aches and pains that were being masked.

Discomfort can also be the result of bad posture. While meditating make sure that you are sitting upright, keeping your head up (imagine your head is being pulled up by a piece of string) and you can even try placing a cushion behind the small of your back.

NINE

TYPES OF MEDITATION

"So what makes a good meditator? The one who meditates."

Allan Lokos

As your interest in meditation increases you will find that there is a literally a sea of various meditation practices. In this book I have included a mix of seven meditation techniques, but how do you know which meditation type is the best?

Firstly, there is no 'best', just the one that works for you in this stage of your life. What typically happens is that when people find a type of meditation that works for them they then become 'evangelists' for that type of meditation. The problem is that what works for one may not connect with another.

Scientists generally class meditation types into two main categories based on the way they focus attention: focused attention and open monitoring. Let's take a look at these two broad categories and the meditation types associated with them.

Focused Attention Meditation

In this category of meditation ones attention is focused upon a single object during the whole meditation session. The object of attention may be the breath, a mantra, visualization, a part of the body, external objects, etc. Some examples of these meditation types would be: Loving Kindness Meditation, Mantra Meditation, TM, and Body Scan's to name a few.

Loving Kindness Meditations is derived from the Buddhist traditions (Tibetan). In this meditation practice one seeks to develop positive emotions through compassion, self-acceptance, and empathy. This meditation is practiced by generating feelings of kindness and benevolence towards yourself and others. You start by generating these feelings for yourself, then a good friend, then a neutral person followed by a difficult person and finally for the entire universe.

Mantra Meditations come from Hindu traditions and use a word, such as 'OM', as the focal point. Some people teach that the word is not important, as it is just a tool to focus the mind, and others hold that the word and its correct pronunciation are essential, as the word creates a mental vibration that allows the mind to experience deeper levels of awareness. Meditation beads are usually used to assist in keeping count (there are 108 beads) as the mantra is repeated 108 or 1008 times.

Transcendental Meditation (TM) is a specific form of Mantra Meditation introduced by Maharishi Mahesh Yogi in 1955 and was made famous when Maharishi became guru to celebrities such as The Beatles and The Beach Boys. It is a widely practiced form of meditation with over five million practitioners world-wide. This is an expensive form of meditation as the only way to learn it is from one of TM's licensed instructors. There is a much cheaper version of it called Natural Stress Relief, which was developed by an ex-TM instructor.

Open Monitoring Meditation

In open monitoring meditations all aspects of ones experience are monitored without judgment or attachment. Examples of these types of meditation are Mindfulness Meditation and Taoist Meditation.

Mindfulness Meditations is a Westernized versions of Buddhist forms of Zen and Vipassana Meditation. One of the main influencers for Mindfulness in the West is John Kabat-Zinn who developed the Mindfulness-Based Stress Reduction program (MBSR) in 1979 and it is now offered in over 200 medical centers, hospitals and clinics around the world. In Mindfulness Meditation the aim is to pay attention to what is going on in the present moment without losing oneself in anything that arises. Practicing mindfulness is also encouraged in ones daily activities so that one isn't living in 'automatic mode'.

Taoist Meditation comes from Chinese traditions and it's purpose is to quiet the body and mind, unify the body and spirit, find inner peace and harmony with the Tao (nature). One simply allows all thoughts and sensations to arise and fall without any engagement with the thoughts.

I have just scratched the surface of the meditation types that are available. I trust that this chapter has given you the basics so you can have an idea of what is out there and so that you can know what type of meditation that you are practicing.

TEN

FAQ'S

"Judge a man by his questions rather than by his answers."

Voltaire

As you continue along your meditative journey you may find that you have a few questions. In this chapter I will answer six of the most common questions about meditation.

How Often and How Long Should I Meditate For?

You may have noticed that throughout this book I haven't mentioned a length of time (except in the deep breathing section). Too often we get hung up on what we 'should' be accomplishing. Just relax and start out with what works for you. You might start with three minutes or five or ten. Pretty soon you'll just naturally want to go longer and time will fly by.

You'll probably find that a lot of places suggest you meditate for twenty minutes. I have found it much for helpful for those starting out to go for three, five or ten minutes. The important thing is to doing what will work for you right now in this space and season in your life. It is far better to meditate daily for five minutes than to meditate once a week for twenty minutes.

Just remember not to get caught up in the 'shoulds'.

How long should one bath for? You see what I mean? Just do what works for you.

As for the time of day, many people find morning and evenings a great time to meditate. But once again, just do what works for you.

One tip however, is that it is usually not the best idea to meditate straight after a meal.

You can also break up your meditations throughout the day. Once again, just do what works for you. This may also change in the various seasons and stages of your life.

The most important thing is to find a time that works for you and schedule this and make it a regular routine.

Charles Duhigg in his book The Power of Habit gives a great action plan on how to form habits that stick. MIT researchers identified that at the core of our habits are simple neurological loops. These loops are made up of cues (location, time, emotional state, other people or an immediately preceding action), routines and rewards.

Once you've figured out your habit loop – you've identified the reward driving the behavior, the cue triggering it, and the routine itself – you can begin to shift the unwanted behavior. You can then change to a better routine by planning for the cue, and choosing a behavior that delivers the reward that you are craving.

It's a great read, and can be a game changer in your life. You can view the book at http://futurepastpodcast.com/meditation-resources/

How Do I Know When I am Getting Better at Meditating?

There is no such thing as good or bad meditation, but through continued practice and attention to your object of focus, the mind becomes sharper, more focused and more alert.

Which Meditation Type Is Right For Me?

There is no 'right' meditation practice, just the one that works for you at that time. Over time you may outgrow a particular practice. That's ok. Just keep experimenting.

What Should I Do If I Experience Physical Discomfort?

An unhealthy or weak body may find it difficult to sit in any one position for a long period of time.

Getting up and walking around can alleviate this; try to exercise regularly if this is the case. Having a good stretch before meditating also helps.

Can I Really Learn to Meditate From a Book?

Yes you can, just like multitudes of other people have! You don't have to have personal one on one or group instruction, although some people do connect with this style of learning better. The truth is you can learn to meditate from a sunset, a piece of art, and poetry.

If you are meditating regularly and are thriving, then you know what you need to know.

I have included seven different techniques or practices from various meditation types so that you can discover what works for you. Have fun experimenting!

Is Meditation Religious?

Meditation is a tool, a science and an art.

Most people in the world have already meditated without even realizing it. If you have ever relaxed by looking at a beautiful sunset, allowing your thoughts to quiet down, this is close to meditation.

If you have been reading a book for a while then put it down to take a break and just sat there quietly and peacefully for a few minutes without thinking, this is close to meditation.

Meditation is of itself non-religious. It can, and is used in various religious practices, but it is not itself a religion or tied to any religion. It is a practice of good health.

ELEVEN

FURTHER RESOURCES

"Be here now. Be someplace else later. Is that so complicated?"

David M Bader

Well done on making it this far! Hopefully you have already given meditation a go. I'm sure you were surprised by the results. And the best thing is that you didn't have to get all 'woo-woo' to experience it.

As a gift for making it this far in the book I'd like to give you a free guided audio meditation. I'd also love to be able to stay in touch with you and let you know when new books are released. Simply go to http://futurepastpodcast.com/get-your-free-meditation-bonus/

As you are beginning your journey it can be difficult to know what other quality resources are out there. To make it easier for you I will list some below:

Books

The 5-Minute Meditator by Eric Harrison

Eric Harrison is one of Australia's most experienced meditation teachers. He has taught over 20 000 people at his meditation centre in Perth.

Eric has found that while many of his students enjoyed the benefits of meditation that less than half of them continued because they were too busy. Eric has written this book for those who have 'no time to meditate'… the one's who need it most!

The book is an easy read and filled with easy to apply meditations that focus on: your body and breath; your senses; and including activities such as cooking, housework and driving into your meditations.

How I Rescued My Brain by David Roland

As a forensic psychologist, David Roland often saw the toughest and most heart breaking cases. The emotional trauma had begun to take its toll – and then global financial crisis hit leaving his family facing financial ruin.

Join David on an incredible journey and learn how mindfulness and meditation helped him back to recovery.

It's an easy read and I can highly recommend the book.

Wherever You Go, There You Are by Jon Kabat-Zinn

This is a national bestseller. In the book Jon talks about mindfulness meditation and how you can apply it. Although Jon is not a Buddhist he does fill you in on how the Eastern mind-sets which I found quite interesting.

Go to http://futurepastpodcast.com/meditation-resources/ to purchase or borrow the books on Amazon.

Binaural Beats

Binaural Beats are said to massage your brain and help induce relaxation, meditation, creativity and other desirable mental states.

The effect on your brainwaves depends on the difference in frequencies of the tones sent to each ear: for example if 300 Hz was played in one ear and 310 Hz was played in the other.

I personally use binaural beats for my power naps, but I have been recommended to use them for meditation.

They can be purchased and found free on the web and in app stores. Try a free version and see what you think.

Apps For Your Phone

Calm

I have personally used Calm. It is an excellent guided meditative app for beginners without any woo-woo. It is available on PC, Android and IOS. It's a free app and you can pay to open extra features. You can find them at http://www.calm.com

Headspace

Headspace is another great app with heaps of meditation techniques and applications. The Take 10 program is free (and really brilliant with great animations that explain things very well) but other than that you'll need to subscribe for US$12.95 a month. You can check them out at https://www.headspace.com

Lucent

This is a meditation app that is not guided. It gives you an opportunity to choose your mood before and after your meditation session. It also gives you an opportunity to journal any insights, what you're grateful for and an action that you will take today. You can check out the website at http://www.lucentapp.com

Breathe2Relax

Breathe2Relax can help with your Deep Breathing exercises. It is a free app. You can find them at http://breathe2relax.soft112.com

TWELVE

IN CLOSING

"Accept what life offers you and try to drink from every cup. All wines should be tasted; some should only be sipped, but with others, drink the whole bottle."
- Paulo Coelho

I want to thank you for choosing this book.

In this book you have learned about the incredible benefits of meditation and the mind-set that is needed. You've also learned about the centrepiece – breath. This is a book that is designed to get you meditating, not just learning about it. I trust that you'll enjoy trying out the four deep breathing and seven meditation techniques.

Hopefully I have also forewarned you that the meditative road can get rocky. I trust that being forewarned of the five most common obstacles will equip you to overcome these obstacles. In these times when the journey seems difficult, it would be a wise idea to fill yourself with encouragement through reading and listening to meditation resources.

Another way to ensure your success is to share what you have been learning with others. Not only do you get to add value to another's life, but you will also be able to encourage one another when the going gets tough. As Stephen S. Wise says, *"An unshared life is not living. He who shares does not lessen, but greatens, his life."*

Finally, your meditative journey is a highly personal one, so try not to compare your journey with anyone else's. We all have our own path to travel. As long as you are developing in your sense of presence, and you are continually returning to your focus, you will find your mind becoming more alert, creative and focused.

This is just the beginning of your meditation journey. May your journey see you live a centered, connected and successful life.

ABOUT THE AUTHOR

Clive Smit is an entrepreneur, speaker and writer. He is the founder of the Future Past Podcast, an on-line mentoring hub for those who want to develop their personal growth and leadership. Previously he served as a pastor in four churches across two continents (South Africa and New Zealand) for seventeen years. He has also worked as a business development manager in the NZ recruitment industry.
Clive is married to Selina and they have four children.

You can learn more about Clive by visiting http://futurepastpodcast.com

www.ingramcontent.com/pod-product-compliance
Lightning Source LLC
Chambersburg PA
CBHW021337290326
41933CB00038B/959